The Autoimmune Paleo Plan

A Revolutionary Protocol To
Rapidly Decrease Inflammation and
Balance Your Immune System

by

Anne Angelone

TABLE OF CONTENT

ISBN-13: 978-1483973517
ISBN-10: 1483973514

Disclaimer

This program manual is not intended to provide medical advice or to take the place of medical advice and treatment from your personal physician

Readers are advised to consult their own doctors or other qualified health professionals regarding the treatment of medical conditions

The author, shall not be held liable or responsible for any misunderstanding or misuse of the information contained in this program manual or for any loss, damage, or injury caused or alleged to be caused directly or indirectly by any treatment, action, or application of any food or food source discussed in this program manual

The statements in this program manual have not been evaluated by the U.S Food and Drug Administration

This information is not intended to diagnose, treat, cure, or prevent any disease.

To request permission for reproduction or inquire about consulting about autoimmunity, please contact:

Anne Angelone, Licensed Acupuncturist

website: www.anneangelone.com

INTRODUCTION

You are probably reading this right now because you suffer from an autoimmune condition and know from personal experience that certain foods contribute to your body discomfort and inflammation. You are likely in need of a reliable plan that inspires you, or perhaps you are seeking to refine your current dietary approach. Perhaps you'd like to grasp the depth of the conversation going on between you and the food you eat.

I see patients with various autoimmune conditions such as RA, Ankylosing Spondylitis, Hashimoto's Thyroiditis, Psoriasis, Eczema, Ulcerative Colitis, and Celiac at my clinic in San Francisco.

Without exception, autoimmune patients are in need of an effective anti-inflammatory diet and lifestyle plan to calm down and balance their overactive immune systems.

The following are some general concerns of autoimmune patients:

1. Knowing what to eat and what to avoid.
2. Resolving dysbiosis, SIBO, and repairing leaky gut.
3. Cooling inflammation and oxidative stress.
4. Balancing the immune system.
5. Reducing stress and improving sleep.

Current discoveries in the field of immunity confirm that certain foods and bacteria irritate the mucosal lining of the gut and contribute both to intestinal permeability (aka leaky gut) and the autoimmune response, generally experienced as a flare-up, attack, or an exacerbation of symptoms.

The goal of The Autoimmune Paleo Plan is to fix your leaky gut and eliminate food and bacterial triggers to autoimmune reactions with the ultimate intention of decreasing your flare-ups and severity of autoimmune attacks.

For anyone with an autoimmune disease, eliminating known inflammatory foods from your diet, resolving dysbiosis, and healing the mucosal lining of the small intestine are the keys to optimal health and balanced immunity.

It may be a new lens through which to consider how poorly digested foods continue to irritate the lining of your gut, feed your yeast and bacterial overgrowths, trigger autoantibody responses, and may set the stage for you to express your genetic tendency to autoimmunity. Yet, since 80% of your immune system is in your gut, you probably already know that digestive health is of paramount importance in healing autoimmune conditions.

The Autoimmune Paleo Plan is designed to rapidly reduce inflammation and heal intestinal permeability via specific dietary interventions. To calm down the immune/inflammatory response and allow the gut to heal, you will need to remove the major offending foods: eggs, grains, alcohol, nightshades, nuts, seeds, legumes, and dairy for at least 30 days.

Some will need to continue for several months to a year.

While on the The Autoimmune Paleo Plan, it is important to identify and remove overgrowths of yeast, bacteria and parasites that may also be driving your immune/inflammatory response.

The goal is to increase anti-inflammatory and probiotic foods to heal the integrity of the gut lining while simultaneously eliminating the foods that create a low grade immune/inflammatory response, irritate the gut lining, and feed harmful bacteria (which lead to SIBO and dysbiosis). By eliminating the underlying mechanisms that drive inflammation and autoimmunity, you can modulate and bring balance to your overactive immune system.

WHY PALEO?

Paleo is the term used to revere the diet of our pre-agricultural ancestors since it was free of all the grains, processed foods, and sugars that seem to be causing the chronic diseases we face today. In current times, Autoimmune Paleo refers to a lifestyle of embracing an egg, grain, legume, sugar, nightshade, nut/seed, alcohol, and dairy free template of real food nutrition. Based on the fact that these foods are the worst triggers of chronic autoimmune reactions, we can appreciate this stellar dietary template for autoimmune conditions.

WHAT'S THE PLAN?

In essence, you will be utilizing a nutrient dense, plant strong nutritional model designed to remove foods that activate immune responses, irritate the gut lining, and contribute to leaky gut. After 30 days on this plan you should notice significant health benefits. Some will need to continue strictly on this plan for 1 year or longer before any potential food triggers can be introduced.

Exercising for 30 minutes a day is a natural anti-inflammatory and is encouraged for balanced immune function and enhanced sleep.

The Autoimmune Paleo Plan is encouraged as a safe way of decreasing inflammation in your body and helping to heal your leaky gut. Following the "foods to include" list will supply you with nutrient dense, bioavailable vitamins and minerals. Your immune system and genes will be shored up with the right nutrition, allowing your inflamed gut to begin healing.

The dietary emphasis on whole, organic, and nutrient dense foods contributes to optimal digestion and immune function with anti-inflammatory and antioxidant rich fruit and veggies. Blood sugar will stabilize and adrenals will strengthen with lots of minerals and amino acids from both protein and veggies. Probiotic and cultured foods will help to reduce intestinal inflammation and provide the nutrients necessary for healthy intestinal micro-flora. Add to that lots of water and herbal teas and you'll be off to a great start.

Other significant considerations for autoimmune conditions include resolving dysbiosis, supporting detoxification and methylation, ramping up glutathione, and increasing regulatory T-cells with vitamin D, probiotics, and fish oils. All of this will go a long way to reduce inflammation and balance the immune system.

Many thanks to leaders who have inspired me in the field of Functional Medicine and Paleo Nutrition: Dr. Eric Gordon, Dr. Tom O'Bryan, Dr. Terry Wahls, Dr. Jeffrey Bland, Dr. Datis Kharrazian, Dr. Alex Vasquez, Dr. Mark Hyman, Dr. Alison Siebecker, Sarah Ballantine, Ph.D., Chris Kresser MS, L.Ac., Diane Sanfilippo, BS, NC, Robb Wolf, Nora Gegaudas, Dr. Loren Cordain, Mat Lalonde Ph.D, Dr. Alessio Fasano, Elaine Gottschall, Natasha Campbell McBride, Stephen Wright and Jordan Reasoner.

The Autoimmune Paleo Plan is inspired by successful treatment outcomes in applying Nutrigenomics, Functional Medicine, Dr. Kharrazian's RepairVite program and the Paleo Autoimmune Protocol. Many thanks to Elaine Fawcett and Sarah Ballantyne, PhD. for help in writing, editing and getting the word out about nutrition for autoimmune conditions.

What triggers autoimmunity?

We now know that genes and the environment are not the only two predisposing factors for autoimmunity. It is now recognized that our genes and environmental triggers interact only due to a breach in the intestinal barrier.

Leaky gut is now recognized as the breached barrier through which our genes and environmental triggers interact and is thus considered the third predisposing factor that sets the stage for autoimmune reactions.

What exactly is leaky gut?

Intestinal permeability (aka leaky gut) refers to the opening of the mucosal lining in the small intestine, which allows food, yeast, and bacteria in the intestines to interact with the immune system.

Dr. Alessio Fasano, of the Maryland Center for Celiac Research, has demonstrated that intestinal permeability or "leaky gut" plays a significant role in triggering most autoimmune conditions.

Considering this connection, healing a leaky gut may prove to be the key to halting the progression of autoimmunity. The questions to keep in mind in terms of preventing autoimmune reactions are:

1. What triggers leaky gut?

2. Can I identify and remove gut irritants?

3. Is there a way to hack my genes to shut down the inflammatory response and allow for disease free expression?

How Do I Know If I Have Leaky Gut Syndrome?

These days you can do a test to find out yet some obvious signs of leaky gut include gas, bloating, poor digestion, multiple food and chemical sensitivities, gut pain, and inflammation. Some not so obvious signs of leaky gut (which manifest outside the small intestine) include decreased mental clarity (aka brain fog), headache, depression, allergies, eczema, body aches, and fatigue.

Fixing a leaky gut is definitely a priority for autoimmune conditions.

Intestinal permeability has been found in connection with the following autoimmune diseases: Ankylosing Spondylitis, Apthous stomatitis, asthma, autism, autoimmune gastritis, autoimmune hepatitis, Behcet's Syndrome, Celiac disease, Depression, Dermatitis Herpetiformis, Type 1 Diabetes, Eczema, Gut migraine in children, and Hashimoto's Thyroiditis. Leaky gut is also frequently seen in asthma, psoriasis, and nearly all of the currently so called idiopathic juvenile arthritides.

What Triggers leaky gut?

TEN TRIGGERS OF LEAKY GUT

Although the causes of leaky gut can be ambiguous, Datis Kharrazian, DHSc, DC, MS has identified 10 factors that contribute to leaky gut:

1. Diet:

Most people blame poor diet, and rightly so, as many popular foods can damage the gut. Gluten in particular is associated with gut damage. Dairy, lectins, processed foods, excess sugar, and fast foods are also common culprits. Excess alcohol is another gut saboteur.

2. Medications:

Certain medications increase the risk of leaky gut. They include corticosteroids, antibiotics, antacids, NSAIDS, and some medications for arthritis. Some medications may also contain gluten as a filler.

3. Infections:

An overgrowth of H. pylori, a bacterium in the stomach, can cause ulcers and leaky gut. Overgrowth of other harmful bacteria (SIBO), yeast infections, parasitic infections, and intestinal viruses can also cause leaky gut.

4. Stress:

Chronic stress raises the adrenal hormone, cortisol, which degrades the gut lining and contributes to leaky gut.

5. Hormone imbalances:

The gut depends on proper hormone levels for good health. When estrogen, progesterone, testosterone, or thyroid hormones are deficient or out of balance, this imbalance can contribute to leaky gut.

6. Autoimmune conditions:

We often think of leaky gut contributing to autoimmune diseases such as Hashimoto's hypothyroidism, rheumatoid arthritis, or psoriasis. While this may be true, sometimes other factors can trigger an autoimmune condition, including toxic exposures or stress. In these cases, the autoimmune condition can be the cause of leaky gut and managing autoimmunity is a strategy to improving leaky gut.

7. Industrial food processing:

The food processing industry uses a variety of methods that can increase intestinal inflammation and leaky gut. These include deamidating wheat to make it water soluble, high-heat processing (glycation) of sugars, and adding excess sugar to processed foods.

8. Environmental toxins:

We are surrounded by toxins in our environment. Some of these toxins have been found to break down immune barriers like the gut. One way to shore up your defense against environmental toxins is to make sure your body is sufficient in glutathione, the body's primary antioxidant.

9. Vitamin D deficiency:

Sufficient vitamin D is vital to good health and helps preserve gut integrity.

10. Poor glutathione status:

Glutathione is the body's primary antioxidant and is necessary to defend and repair the gut lining. Poor diet and lifestyle factors deplete glutathione.

These are just some of the factors identified by Dr. Kharrazian in the scientific literature as contributing to leaky gut.

Since these triggers may degrade the mucosal lining of the gut and lead to autoimmune reactions, patients are encouraged to decrease stress, balance their hormones, resolve SIBO and dysbiosis, avoid food sensitivities, and modulate the immune sytem.

The plan is always to remove leaky gut triggers, resolve dysbiosis, and restore a healthy intestinal barrier to reduce any systemic inflammatory reactions that are driving auto-antibody attacks (i.e. your autoimmune condition).

Along with the autoimmune dietary template, L-Glutamine, zinc, DGL, aloe, and probiotic foods can help to support the integrity of the gut lining.

SIBO and Dysbiosis

Beyond removing inflammatory foods and healing a leaky gut, patients with autoimmune conditions need to investigate small intestine bacterial overgrowth and dysbiosis that may contribute to leaky gut and the auto-antibody response. Dysbiosis refers to an overgrowth of yeast, bacteria, and/or parasites located in the gastrointestinal tract.

Small Intestine Bacterial Overgrowth (SIBO) is now being considered as a significant yet overlooked cause of IBS. SIBO can cause nausea, gas, bloating, diarrhea, and/or constipation. Bacterial toxins from SIBO (called lipopolysaccharides) can impair absorption, and result in nutrient deficiencies, fat malabsorption, food intolerances, poorly functioning digestive enzymes, leaky gut, and the auto-antibody response (i.e. autoimmune reactions).

What Causes Bacterial Overgrowth?

The entire gastrointestinal (GI) tract contains bacteria, both good and bad. The small intestine contains bacteria different from that of the large intestine. In the case of SIBO, the small intestine contains too much bacteria, and these bacteria more closely resemble the bacteria of the colon. These bacteria consume sugars and carbohydrates, producing large amounts of gas. FODMAP malabsorption (see below), inadequate dietary fiber, hypochlorhydria (decreased stomach acid), and pancreatic enzyme deficiency set the stage for inadequate digestion in susceptible individuals and contribute to poorly digested carbs which in turn feed bacteria in the small intestine. Bacterial endotoxins, called lipopolysaccharadies, further contribute to leaky gut and the inflammatory fire that needs to be extinguished.

To correct the problem, a no grain, low starch diet is imperative and suggested in the Autoimmune Paleo Plan. Some may need to completely restrict allowable starches like yams and sweet potatoes and go for a «no starch» version of the Autoimmune Paleo Plan to completely starve SIBO (i.e. no yams, sweet potatoes, dense carbs) Others may also need to use antibiotics and/or botanical antimicrobials (dysbiotics) along with extra hydrochloric acid and digestive enzyme supplementation.

SIBO CAUTION FOODS IN THE AIP:

Parsnips, yams, jicama, kohlrabi, okra, sweet potato, taro, plantain, Jerusalem artichoke, parsnips, lotus root, cassava root, manioc, tapioca, yucca.

SIBO CAUTION FOODS *(NOT IN THE AIP)*:

Chestnuts, bitter gourd.

FODMAPS

FODMAPs:

Describe short-chain carbohydrates found in many common foods. FODMAPs stands for Fermentable Oligo-, Di- and Mono-saccharides, and Polyols (sugar alcohols).

FODMAP intolerance can tip you off to the possibility of having small intestine bacterial overgrowth. If poorly digested, these carbs will feed bad bacteria (SIBO), which in turn produce methane and hydrogen gas that can cause bloating, cramping, burping, gas, diarrhea and other bowel problems that generally get diagnosed as IBS. If these bacterial overgrowths remain untreated, they may contribute to leaky gut and the inflammatory/immune response.

If you have IBS symptoms and are not improving on the *standard* Paleo Autoimmune Protocol, the best way to check for *FODMAP* sensitivity would be to remove these foods for at least 30 days and then reintroduce them and check for *SIBO* if there is no change. If you desire to reintroduce these foods, make sure you have resolved the root cause of your FODMAP intolerance to avoid symptoms.

FODMAPs in the autoimmune protocol:

Apples, artichokes, apricots, cherries, pears, plum, persimmon, nectarines, peaches, pluots, artichoke, asparagus, cabbage, garlic, leeks, okra, onions, radicchio, avocado, beet root, broccoli, Brussels sprouts, mushrooms, butternut squash, pumpkin, cauliflower, celery, fennel bulb, mushrooms, sauerkraut, dried coconut, coconut flour, coconut milk, coconut cream, coconut butter, honey, grapes, dried fruits, blackberries, apricots, shallots.

FODMAPs *(not in the AIP)*:

pistachios, almonds, hazelnuts, cheese,milk, yogurt, green peas, chicory, fructo-oligosaccharide, inulin,prebiotics, onion and garlic powder, gums, carrageenan, sorbitol, mannitol, xylitol, isomalt, port wine, beer, agave, fruit juices, tomato sauce and paste, chicory root, onion powder, garlic powder.

FOOD SENSITIVITIES

Immunogenic or Allergenic

Immunogenic reactions to foods are inflammatory responses, which activate part of the immune system but will not cause an IgE allergy response or anaphylactic shock. This causes a low grade inflammatory response or an IgG reaction. This means that you are sensitive, rather than allergic. There are many possible foods that may be creating this response in your immune system. Common foods that create this response include gluten, dairy, corn, soy, and nightshade vegetables. With a smoldering and undetected IgG response, along with a leaky gut, the potential for the autoantibody response also increases as your immune system is now on high surveillance in order to attack the similar protein structures of the offending foods. During the fight, your immune system may confuse your joint tissue or your thyroid as the offending food protein. Even though it's trying to do its job, think of it as the immune system coping with an unnecessary burden that can be dropped by eliminating these foods.

SALICYLATE SENSITIVITY:

Salicylate sensitivity has the potential to create more inflammation in the body and has been linked to IBS, Crohn's and Colitis. High salicylate foods have also been linked to the following symptoms: itchy skin, hives or rashes, stomach pain, nausea and/or diarrhea, asthma and other breathing difficulties e.g. persistent cough, headaches, swelling of hands, feet, tissue swelling of the eyelids, face and/or lips (angioedema), changes in skin color, fatigue, sore, itchy, puffy or burning eyes, nasal congestion or sinusitis, memory loss and poor concentration (linked to ADHD), ringing in the ears, depression and anxiety.

HIGH SALICYLATE FOODS IN THE AIP:

Berries, apricot, avocado, blackberry, cherries, plum/prune, green olives, endive, gherkin, radish, tangelo, tangerine, water chestnut, coconut oil, olive oil, all dried fruits, honey, date, grape, guava, orange, pineapple.

High Salicylate Foods that are not in the autoimmune protocol to consider if reintroducing to your diet: Almond, all nightshades: peppers, eggplant, tomato, chili etc.

HIGH HISTAMINE FOODS

Those who have salicylate intolerance may also have histamine intolerance. Like FODMAP intolerance, Histamine intolerance may tip you off to SIBO and/or dysbiotic bacteria. When these bacteria secrete histamine, the enzyme system that breaks down histamine gets overwhelmed which results in allergic symptoms similar to salicylate intolerance: nasal congestion, rashes, abdominal cramping, nausea, asthma, runny nose, itchy skin, watery eyes, hives, fatigue, headaches, irritability, heartburn, angioedema. Many of the foods that are high in salicylates are also high in histamines.

High Histamine Foods in the AIP:

Oranges, grapefruit, lemons, lime, sauerkraut, bacon spinach, cinnamon, vinegar, shellfish, leftover meat, vinegar pickles, sauerkraut, kombucha, spinach, berries, cloves, dried fruit.

High Histamine Foods that are not in the autoimmune protocol to consider if reintroducing to your diet: Eggs, aged cheese, tomatoes, eggplant, alcohol, lunch meats, sausage, chocolate, cocoa, colas, tea, relishes, ketchup, dairy based yogurt, buttermilk and kefir, fermented soy products, tomatoes, ketchup, tomato sauces, artificial food colors, preservatives, chili powder, anise, nutmeg, curry powder, cayenne.

HIGH OXALATE FOODS

Foods that are high in oxalates can contribute to pain and inflammation.

High Oxalate Foods in the autoimmune protocol:

Sweet potatoes, endive, asparagus, Brussels sprouts, cucumbers, celery and beets, chard, beet greens.

High Oxalate Foods that are not in the autoimmune protocol to consider if reintroducing to your diet: eggplant, almonds, walnuts, cashews, pecans, sunflower, sesame, peanut, pinto beans, black beans, soy beans, rye, millet, oats, corn, potatoes, tea, coffee, beer.

GOITROGENIC FOODS:

For Graves or Hashimoto's patients who still have a thyroid and are not on thyroid medications, consider only moderate quantities of goitrogenic foods including raw broccoli, cabbage, bok choy, Brussels sprouts, cauliflower, collard, radishes, spinach, pears, peaches, and strawberries. Cooking reduces goitrogens; fermentation increases them.

Support Your Immune System

GOING BEYOND TH1 AND TH2

When we manage an autoimmune disease in functional medicine, we identify why the immune system is imbalanced, and then work to restore that balance. The pro-inflammatory side of the immune system (also called "TH-1") responds immediately to an invader in the body. The anti-inflammatory side of the immune system ("TH-2") has a delayed response and produces antibodies to an invader. These antibodies tag the invader so that if it shows up again, the immune system can respond more quickly. In a healthy person, these two systems work in balance. However, in the person with an autoimmune disease, one of these systems has become overly dominant.

This polarity between TH-1 and TH-2 underlies autoimmune conditions, and we use nutritional therapies to help restore balance. This helps tame inflammation and autoimmune disease.

THE NEW IMMUNE PLAYER: TH-17

Studies have increasingly spotlighted another important player in the immune system called TH-17. While appropriate expression of TH-17 is important for immune defense, over-activation of TH-17 plays a key role in autoimmune disease and chronic inflammatory disease. When it comes to quenching flare-ups, TH-17 is our newest target. Since TH17 activates Nuclear Factor Kappa Beta, if we can remove triggers and break the cycle of inflammation with specific nutrients and botanicals, we can go a long way to decreasing inflammation.

Immune Regulation

SUPPORTING REGULATORY T-CELLS

Curcumin, glutathione, vitamin D, and fish oil work by supporting "regulatory T cells" (aka TH3 cells). These cells do what they say—they regulate the activity of TH-17, TH-1, and TH-2, keeping all the facets of the immune system in check. When they don't work efficiently, the immune system can tip out of balance, thus promoting inflammation and autoimmunity. Other specific compounds that successfully support regulatory T-cells include vitamin A, non-dairy probiotic strains, and nutrients that boost activity of our master antioxidant glutathione, plus nutrients that act on nitric oxide pathways as recommended above.

GLUTATHIONE

Glutathione is the body's primary antioxidant and is necessary to defend

and repair the gut lining. Although the body naturally makes and recycles glutathione, modern life can overwhelm this system, depleting us of this vital compound. When glutathione is low the body is more vulnerable to disease and damage, and your risk for disease rises.

Glutathione as a supplement is not well absorbed by the digestive tract. Fortunately, many nutritional compounds act as building blocks to glutathione, and can help raise and maintain its levels inside and outside of cells. You can also obtain glutathione intravenously.

Below are some of many nutritional compounds that have been shown to boost glutathione levels.

- N-acetyl-cysteine is a very bioavailable building block to glutathione.
- Alpha lipoic acid helps recycle glutathione already in the cells.
- Milk thistle boosts glutathione.
- Methylation nutrients--methyl folate (5-MTHF), methyl B6 (P5P) and methyl B12 (methylcobalmin)--are methyl forms of B vitamins can help boost glutathione production and recycling.
- Selenium helps the body produce and recycle glutathione.
- Vitamin C help increase glutathione levels.

Diet and lifestyle factors can also affect your glutathione levels. Sulfur-rich foods such as garlic, onions, broccoli, kale, collards, cabbage, cauliflower, and watercress can help boost glutathione. Exercise also boosts glutathione; get aerobic exercise daily (such as walking) and strength training two to three times a week.

One of the most important ways to maintain your glutathione levels is to reduce stress on your body.

Glutathione's job is to protect the cells, whether it's from an autoimmune disease, sleep deprivation, or the toxic ingredients in scented detergents and fabric softeners. Healthy glutathione levels reduce your risk of developing chronic and autoimmune disease as well as food and chemical sensitivities. It is also an excellent anti-aging compound.

The following are some strategies to prevent depletion of glutathione.

- Find out what your food intolerances are and remove those foods from your diet. Many people are not aware that they are intolerant to common foods, such as bread or cheese. The autoimmune protocol, which is essentially an elimination diet, or a lab test can help you determine which foods are stressing your immune system and taxing glutathione reserves.

- Eat an all-natural, whole foods diet as suggested here. Processed foods and fast foods contain chemical additives, genetically altered foods, antibiotics, hormones, excess sugar, and other ingredients that are stressful to the body and deplete glutathione.

- Get enough sleep. Sleep deprivation is very stressful. If you have issues sleeping, it is often secondary to something else.

- Manage your autoimmune disease. An autoimmune or chronic disease, such as Hashimoto's hypothyroidism, rheumatoid arthritis, or diabetes keeps the immune system on overdrive and damages tissue, depleting glutathione.

- Reduce your exposure to toxins and pollutants. Many common environmental chemicals are toxic to the body. They are found in shampoos, body products, household cleaners, lawn care products, and so on. We have enough to deal with in terms of pollutants in air and water, minimize your exposure to them in the home.

- EMFs are a source of "electrical pollution." Cell phones, computers, WiFi, and other electronics are stressful to the body and exposure should be minimized.

VITAMIN D

Vitamin D is a corner stone to good health, however research shows many people do not get enough from sunlight and diet alone. In general, we spend most of our lives indoors, wear sunscreen when outside, and don't eat a vitamin D-rich diet.

More than 40 percent of the population and 60 percent of children are estimated deficient. Living at a northern latitude, obesity, and aging also increase the risk for deficiency. One study found 60 percent of postmenopausal to be deficient in vitamin D.

If you suffer from an autoimmune disease or other chronic illness, boosting vitamin D levels (cholecalciferol) will help you outpace and prevent disease by supporting regulatory T-cell production. Besides supplementing with a pill, you can get Vitamin D from cod liver oil, herring, trout, salmon, halibut, mushrooms, beef liver and sunshine.

OMEGA 3 FATTY ACIDS

Omega 3 fatty acids also support regulatory T-cells. Besides supplementing with fish oil capsules, you can increase your intake of beneficial anti-inflammatory omega 3's by include foods in your diet like salmon, sardines, tuna, mackerel and grass fed meats.

PROBIOTICS

Besides supplementing with non-dairy probiotics, you can replenish good flora in the gut by including foods like sauerkraut, coconut yogurt, kimchee, kombucha and coconut kefir.

VITAMIN A

You can obtain Vitamin A from liver, sweet potatoes, carrots, dark leafy greens, butternut squash, pumpkin, cod liver oil and Vitamin E from basil, oregano, olives, spinach.

Hacking Gene Expression

NUTRIGENOMICS

For all autoimmune reactions, the goal is the suppression of the inflammatory response. Nutrigenomics is an exciting field of nutritional science that looks at how food/nutrients can regulate inflammatory gene expression and thus suppress the inflammatory response. The process of silencing inflammatory gene suppression via certain nutrients is called DNA methylation.

METHYLATION

Many patients with autoimmune conditions are genetically predisposed to methylation defects and need to consider supplementing with folate, vitamin B6, and vitamin B12 to ensure proper methylation. Daily green smoothies will supply a good source of these methylation factors and are encouraged. Methylation nutrients–methyl folate (5-MTHF), methyl B6 (P5P) and methyl B12 (methylcobalmin)–are methyl forms of B vitamins can help boost glutathione production and recycling.

Hacking Inflammation

SILENCING NUCLEAR FACTOR KAPPA BETA

NFKB is a transcription factor that stimulates pro-inflammatory gene expression. When we investigate what activates NFKB, we can appreciate why it's important to treat the root cause of inflammation.

Leaky gut, dysbiosis, SIBO, food sensitivities, stress, and viruses can all activate NFKB and lead to an increased expression of pro-inflammatory genes that code for the production of inflammatory cytokines. Of course the goal is to root out the triggering source of this inflammatory response by eliminating poorly digested proteins, resolving dysbiosis, SIBO, and healing up your leaky gut.

Along the way we can modulate NFKB with botanicals like curcumin.

SUPPORTING NITRIC OXIDE SYSTEM PATHWAYS

Autoimmune reactions increase the output of cytokines that acitvate inducible nitric oxide synthase (iNOS), which in turn can contribute to intestinal permeability. Besides healing a leaky gut, it's also important to consider using natural anti-inflammatory and anti-oxidative substances like Huperzine A, Vinpocetine, Adenosine, Alpha-Ketogluteric Acid, and L Acetylcarnitine to aid in dampening inflammation, and tissue repair.

The addition of these remedies, along with eliminating the causes, breaks the cycle of inflammation by decreasing TH17 and inhibiting NFKB. This shuts down the expression of inflammatory genes, their cascade of cytokines, and the expression of your autoimmune condition.

The Autoimmune Paleo Plan

GUIDELINES:

Do's

- Eat organic, pastured, grass fed animal protein and wild fish.
- Eat carbohydrates from fruits and vegetables.
- Eat fat from avocados, coconut, and olive oil.
- Eat low glycemic fruits and non-starchy vegetables.
- Eat fermented foods like sauerkraut, coconut kefir, and yogurt.
- Eat Superfoods on a daily basis.
- Eat fiber from fruits and vegetables.
- Eat colorful veggies.
- Drink 8 glasses of water including veggie or bone broth daily.
- Exercise every day, preferably for 30 minutes.
- Meditate for at least 5 minutes per day.
- Take daily detox baths with Epsom salts, and baking soda.
- Drink green smoothies daily.
- Get 7-9 hours of sleep.
- Consider digestive enzymes, hydrochloric acid, and apple cider vinegar.

Don'ts:

- No grains at all.
- No dairy products
- No genetically modified organism (GMO) foods.
- No processed foods.
- No refined sugars.
- No wine or alcohol.
- No cereals or grain like seeds.
- No smoked or salted foods.
- No ibuprofen, aspirin or acetaminophen, naproxen.
- No legumes (e.g. peanuts, beans, lentils, peas, and soybeans).
- No nuts, seeds or seed based spices.
- No nightshade vegetables.
- No fruit juices.
- No skipping meals.

A word about caution foods on the autoimmune protocol food lists:

Generally speaking, these foods are either immunogenic, hard to digest, likely to feed gut bacterial overgrowths, dysbiosis, and/or contribute to blood sugar imbalance. If your gut immunity is strong (no overgrowths, no dysbiosis, no food reactions, healthy gut lining), and your blood sugar is balanced, these items may be tolerated in moderation.

Foods to Include:

FRUITS

Apples, apricots, Asian pears, bananas, blueberries, blackberry, boysenberry, cherries, cranberry, figs, grapefruit, kiwi, lemons, limes, melons, nectarine, oranges, peaches, pears, persimmons, plums, pluots, plantains, pomegranate, raspberry, strawberry

Caution: watermelon, mango, pineapple, grapes, dried fruits, dehydrated fruits.

VEGETABLES

Asparagus, arugula, artichoke, avocado, basil, beet, beet greens, broccoli, broccoli rabe, burdock, bok choy, cabbage, carrots, cauliflower, celery, chard, chicory, collards, chard, cucumber, scallion, Jerusalem artichoke, jicama, kale, kohlrabi, lambsquarters, leeks, lettuce, mustard, nettles, okra, onions, purslane, spinach, summer squash, turnips, artichoke hearts, Brussels sprouts, daikon radish, zucchini, fennel root, dandelion greens, red cabbage, green cabbage, Napa cabbage, water chestnuts, watercress, radish, shallot, turnips.

DENSE CARBS

Beets, acorn squash, butternut squash, yams, sweet potato, taro, plantain and lotus root.

FUNGI

Button mushrooms, portabella, oyster, chanterelle, puffball, crimini, etc.

WILD FISH

Salmon, mackerel, herring, halibut, shellfish, oysters, cod, tuna, flounder, sardines, hake, skate, trout, red snapper, etc.

MEAT

Beef, chicken; quail, squab, duck, goose, turkey, Cornish game hen; pasture-raised lamb, pork, buffalo/bison, goat, emu, ostrich, sausage (without fillers or nightshade spices); liver, kidney, heart, organic sliced meats (gluten, sugar free), uncured nitrate/nitrite-free deli meats and bacon from grass-fed/pastured beef/pork.

MILK AND YOGURT

Coconut milk, unsweetened coconut yogurt.

FATS

Extra virgin olive oil, coconut oil, flaxseed, sesame, walnut, hazelnut oil, coconut oil, red palm oil.

Caution: nut and seed based oils: flaxseed oil, sesame oil, walnut oil, hazelnut oil, macadamia nut oil.

COCONUT

Coconut oil, coconut butter, coconut milk, coconut cream, unsweetened coconut yogurt, unsweetened coconut flakes, coconut aminos, coconut kefir.

BEVERAGES

Filtered or distilled water, herbal tea, mineral water, broths, freshly made veggie juice, green smoothies, kombucha, kefir water, coconut kefir.

TEAS

Herbal teas: Peppermint, ginger, lemongrass, spearmint, chamomile, rooibos, lavender, cinnamon, milk thistle.

FERMENTED FOODS

Sauerkraut, pickles, pickled ginger, pickled cucumbers, unsweetened coconut yogurt, unsweetened coconut kefir (without corn or rice-based thickening agents), kombucha, kimchee, kefir water, pickles fermented with salt, beet kvass, lacto-fermented vegetables and fruits such as fermented beets, carrots, and green papaya.

CONDIMENTS

Apple cider vinegar, Balsamic vinegar, coconut vinegar, Red Boat fish sauce and coconut aminos.

HERBS AND SPICES

Turmeric, ginger, rosemary, basil, cilantro, garlic, ginger, lemongrass, peppermint, oregano, parsley, sage, sea, salt, thyme, tarragon, spearmint, marjoram, mace, chives, chamomile, chervil, cinnamon, bay leaves, cloves, dill, horseradish, saffron, sea salt.

Caution: black pepper, allspice, white, green and pink peppercorns, juniper, cardamom, star anise and vanilla bean.

SUGAR SUBSTITUTES

Cinnamon, mint and ginger

Caution: honey, maple syrup, molasses, unrefined cane sugar, and date sugar.

Foods to Eliminate:

NIGHTSHADE VEGETABLES

This includes potatoes (not sweet potatoes), all tomatoes, red and green peppers, chili peppers, eggplants, tomatillos, sweet bell peppers, jalapenos, cayenne, Habanero, Anaheim and Serrano et all peppers.

Avoid chili peppers in dried powders such as paprika, chili powder, curry powder, chili pepper flakes, hot sauces, Tabasco sauces, salsas, goji berries and ashwaganda.

FRUIT

Avoid canned fruits.

Caution: watermelon, mango, pineapple, grapes, dried fruits and dehydrated fruits.

PROCESSED AND CANNED MEATS

Bacon, fatty cuts of lamb, beef, pork, deli meats, smoked/dried/salted meat and fish. Sausages and deli meats with seed-based or nightshade spices.

FISH

Whale, shark, swordfish. Farmed tilapia and catfish quantities should be moderate.

NUTS AND SEEDS

Avoid all nuts and seeds including almonds, Brazil nuts, cashews, chestnuts, hazelnuts, macadamias, pecans, walnuts, pine nuts, pistachios, pumpkin, and sunflower seeds and seed based spices: anise, annatto, black cumin, celery, coriander, cumin, dill, fennel, fenugreek, mustard, nutmeg, poppy, sesame.

DAIRY

Cow and other animal (goat/sheep) milks, cheese, cottage cheese, cream, butter, yogurt, ice-cream, non-dairy creamers, soy milk, whey, butter, cheeses, frozen desserts, mayonnaise.

OILS

Margarine, butter, shortening, any processed hydrogenated oils, peanut oil, mayonnaise.

BEANS AND LEGUMES

Avoid-all beans, black-eyed peas, cashews, chickpeas, lentils, miso, peas, peanuts/peanut butter, soybean and soy products.

FUNGI

Avoid medicinal mushrooms e.g Shiitake, Maitake and Reishi mushrooms.

SOY

Soy milk, soy sauce, tofu, tempeh, soy protein, edamame.

DRINKS

Sodas, fruit juice, alcoholic beverages, coffee, green, black tea, all caffeinated beverages.

CONDIMENTS

Ketchup, relish, soy sauce, BBQ sauce, chutneys, other condiments, baker's and brewer's yeast.

SWEETENERS

Avoid white or brown sugar, high fructose corn syrup, corn syrup, fruit sweeteners, Truvia, maple syrup, agave, brown rice syrup, Splenda, Equal, Nutrasweet, Xylitol, stevia, raw green stevia.

GRAINS

Amaranth, barley, buckwheat, corn including cornmeal and popcorn, millet, oats, oatmeal, quinoa, rice, rye, sorghum, teff, triticale, and wheat including varieties such as spelt, emmer, farro, einkorn, kamut, durum and other forms such as bulgur, cracked wheat and wheat berries.

GRAIN PRODUCTS

Corn tortillas, chips, starch, syrup, noodles, cakes, breads, rolls, muffins, noodles, crackers, cookies, cake, doughnuts, pancakes, waffles, pasta, tortillas, pizza, pita, flat bread.

GRAIN LIKE SUBSTANCES OR PSEUDO-CEREALS

Amaranth, buckwheat, cattail, chia, cockscomb, kañiwa, pitseed, goosefoot, quinoa, and wattleseed (aka acacia seed).

GLUTEN CONTAINING FOODS

BBQ sauce, binders, bouillon, brewer's yeast, cold cuts, condiments, emulsifiers, fillers, gum, hot dogs, hydrolyzed plant and vegetable protein, ketchup, soy sauce, lunch meats, malt, malt flavoring, malt vinegar, matzo, modified food starch, monosodium glutamate, non-dairy creamer, processed salad dressings, seitan, stabilizers, teriyaki sauce, textured vegetable protein.

LEGUMES

Including peas, beans, lentils, soy, and peanuts.

LECTINS

Avoid nuts, beans, soy, potatoes, tomato, eggplant, peppers, peanut oil, peanut butter, soy oil, etc.

DAIRY

All dairy products, including milk cream, cheese, from cows, goats, sheep, etc.

EGGS:

Or foods that contain eggs (e.g mayonnaise).

ALCOHOL

All alcohol.

ALL PROCESSED FOOD

Cured meats, sugar, pre-mixed seasonings and sauces, mayonnaise, mustard, canned foods.

SUGARS

Avoid: white or brown sugar, high fructose corn syrup, corn syrup, fruit sweeteners, Truvia, agave, brown rice syrup, Splenda, Equal, Nutrasweet, Xylitol, stevia, raw green stevia, coconut sugar and palm sugar.

SEED BASED SPICES

Anise, annatto, black cumin, celery, coriander, cumin, dill, fennel, fenugreek, mustard, nutmeg, poppy, sesame, cacao.

BERRY AND FRUIT BASED SPICES

Black pepper, allspice, white, green and pink peppercorns, juniper, cardamom, star anise and vanilla bean.

COFFEE

Remove coffee for 30 days, reintroduce and note reactions.

TEA

Remove caffeinated teas for 30 days, reintroduce and note reactions.

AVOID IMMUNE STIMULANTS

Echinacea purpurea extract, astragalus, ashwaganda, beta glucans, chlorella, glycyrrhiza, licorice root, goldenseal, panax ginseng, grape seed extract, Melissa officinalis (lemon balm), Maitake, Reishi, Shiitake, caffeine, green tea, coffee, lycopene, pine bark extract, willow bark, pycnogenol, genistein, quercetin.

Reintroduction of Foods

Eliminate any foods on the "include" list that you suspect are problematic and do not agree with your constitution. For those not improving on the standard AIP and for those considering reintroduction of foods, it's important to be aware of the foods, herbs and compounds that may contribute to your symptoms and/or autoimmune reactions. These include FODMAPs, starchy foods that contribute to SIBO, foods that create an antibody response (food sensitivities), high oxalate, high histamine and high salicylate foods, cross reactive proteins and immune stimulating herbs and compounds.

CROSS REACTIVE PROTEINS

If you have a known gluten intolerance, as most with autoimmune conditions do, proceed with caution if reintroducing these proteins as they may cause the same antibody/inflammatory reaction as gluten does: dairy proteins (casein, casomorphin, butyrophilin, and whey), oats, brewer/baker's yeast, instant coffee, sorghum, millet, corn, rice and potato.

The Autoimmune Paleo Plan attempts to reduce any of these known food sensitivities in order to reduce the immune/inflammatory response that many patients are getting from these foods.

If symptoms come back after going off the protocol, you can always return to the autoimmune protocol template to rapidly decrease the inflammatory response. Always check with your doctor if you have a flare up of symptoms.

Since reintroduction of foods may cause pronounced reactions, it's important to inform your medical practitioner about your diet and about reintroducing foods and any exacerbation of symptoms.

When reintroducing a food, do so one food at a time, wait 72 hours, note any reactions (headache, joint ache, skin rash, decreased mental clarity etc.), wait until the symptom subsides, then reintroduce the next food.

If symptoms come back after going off the protocol, you can always return to the autoimmune protocol template to rapidly decrease the inflammatory response. Always check with your doctor if you have a flare up of symptoms.

PUTTING THE PLAN INTO ACTION

Essential steps for reversing autoimmunity include clearing out SIBO and dysbiosis, eliminating difficult to digest proteins, avoiding food sensitivities and healing intestinal permeability.

By reducing triggers and fixing the intestinal barrier you will lessen the autoimmune reactions you experience outside of the gut.

Stabilizing blood sugar is also vital to managing autoimmune conditions. A diet high in sugars and refined carbohydrates (such as breads, pastas, pastries, and desserts) creates inflammation and hormonal imbalances that make it difficult to tame an autoimmune condition. Energy crashes, fatigue after meals, excess belly fat, hormonal imbalances, mood swings, and sleep issues are all signs you may have a blood sugar handling disorder, such as hypoglycemia (low blood sugar) or insulin resistance (high blood sugar).

You are encouraged to use the autoimmune protocol template. A serious commitment to the protocol can help set the foundation for halting your autoimmune reactions. Some patients will need to be on this protocol for 30 days, others for several months to one year or longer.

Principles of Functional Medicine for Autoimmune Conditions

Work with a practitioner who can order relevant testing for auto-antibodies, dysbiosis, intestinal permeability, gluten sensitivity, cross reactive proteins, SIBO, lactose and fructose malabsorption.

Once the factors contributing to your autoimmune reactions have been identified, a Functional Medicine practitioner uses a variety of science-backed, non-pharmaceutical approaches to manage health.

These include:

- Adjustments to the diet–to a more appropriate autoimmune diet template.
- Lifestyle changes (such as eating breakfast, proper sleep hygiene, physical activity, or reduction of stress)
- The use of botanicals or nutritional compounds to improve physiological function.
- Other natural medicine approaches customized for the patient based on lab testing.

In Summary, the following may be of paramount importance in halting your autoimmune reactions.

- Supporting regulatory T-cells with: EPA/DHA, Probiotics, Vitamin D, and via supporting Glutathione: NAC, Alpha lipoic acid, L-glutamine, Milk Thistle, Cordyceps, Centella Asiatica, and Selenium.
- Clearing Dysbiosis and SIBO with: antimicrobial, anti-parasitic and/or anti-fungal botanicals and/or pharmaceuticals.
- Supporting the integrity of your gut lining with: L-Glutamine, zinc, DGL, aloe, and probiotic foods.
- Adding digestive enzymes and hydrochloric acid for gas

and bloating.
- Taking a multivitamin, extra magnesium, Vitamin A, C and D.
- Reducing inflammation with curcumin, Huperzine A, Vinpocetine, Adenosine, Alpha GPC, Xanthinol niacinate, and L- acetylcarnitine.
- Supporting detoxification and methylation with folate, B6 and B12.
- Until then remember to:
- Manage your stress
- Cool your inflammation
- Treat your SIBO
- Eat more plants
- Check for FODMAPs
- Eat nutrient dense protein
- Maintain a healthy gut
- Exercise for 30 minutes/day
- Get more sleep
- Stabilize your blood sugar
- Balance your hormones
- Meditate

And most importantly: Have fun!

Delicious Recipes:

COCONUT YOGURT:

6. Heat 1 quart of unsweetened coconut milk to 105F - 110F.
7. Add ¼ teaspoon of yogurt starter and pulse 2x with the blender. You can add more than 1/4 teaspoon per quart if a very firm yogurt is desired.
8. Plug in your yogurt maker and pour the mixture into your yogurt maker container or containers and ferment for 12 hours.
9. Place in refrigerator for 4 hours. Enjoy with blueberries.

GREEN SMOOTHIES:

- 1/2 a bunch dino kale or swiss chard, cut out stalks
- 1/2 inch ginger
- ½ cup blueberries
- 5 cups of water
- Blend for 5 minutes

VEGGIE STEW:

- 1 and ½ cups water, divided
- 4 cups sliced onion
- 2 cups thinly sliced leek
- 1 1/2 cups (1/2-inch-thick) sliced carrots
- 3 cups (1-inch) cubed daikon (about 1 pound)
- 1 bay leaf
- 4 cups (1-inch) cubed zucchini (about 1 1/2 pounds)
- 1/2 teaspoon ground cinnamon
- dash of saffron
- 4 garlic cloves, minced
- 6 cups chopped Swiss chard (about 12 ounces)
- 1/2 cup chopped cilantro

- 2 1/2 teaspoons salt, divided
- 2 tablespoons fresh lemon juice

Add all ingredients to a crock pot or slow cooker. Cook on high heat for 2-3 hours.

FABULOUS KALE CHIPS

Servings: 4.

- 1 large bunch of dino kale, stems removed and leaves chopped
- extra virgin olive oil
- sea salt to taste

Massage Kale with olive oil, sprinkle with sea salt and bake at 350 for 15 min. Let cool and give thanks for a great snack!

GRILL PAN CHICKEN COLLARD WRAP

Servings: 2.

- 6 collard leaves, cut lengthwise into two large pieces (stems removed)
- carrot, cucumber, celery, cut into sticks
- handful of cilantro, whole or chopped
- avocado, sliced into wedges
- 2 organic chicken breasts coated with olive oil thyme and sea salt

Grill chicken, cut into slices and make a wrap with crunchy veggies inside the collard greens.

TRI-TIP STEAK AND ASPARAGUS

Servings: 3

- Tri-tip steak (1 pound)
- 1 head of asparagus
- olive oil
- sea salt
- 2 sprigs of fresh rosemary

Coat everything with olive oil, chopped rosemary, and salt. Grill to perfection.

PALEO PAILLARD

Servings: 5.

5 chicken breasts

salt to taste

1/2 cup coconut flour

3 TB olive or coconut oil

1 cup chicken broth

3 TB capers, drained and rinsed

4 sprigs fresh thyme

Coat chicken with olive oil, and salt. Then dip in coconut flour. Transfer chicken in a single layer to hot skillet and cook chicken cutlets 3 or 4 minutes on each side with capers and thyme. Add broth and cook for 15 minutes. Serve.

BRAISED GREENS

Servings: 4.

- 2 TB coconut or olive oil
- 2 heads of greens
- 1/2 yellow onion, chopped
- 3 garlic cloves, chopped
- 1 1/2 cup vegetable, chicken, or beef stock
- salt to taste
- 2 TB apple cider vinegar

Sautee onion and garlic until golden brown then add greens, salt and vinegar. Cover and let the greens cook down for 20 minutes.

SWEET POTATO FRIES

Servings: 4.

- 3 medium sweet potatoes, washed and peeled
- 3 TB coconut or olive oil
- 1 TB salt or to taste

Coat sweet potatoes with oil, salt. Spread on a baking sheet and bake at 425 for 20 minutes.

CARMELIZED BRUSSELS SPROUTS

Servings: 4.

- 1 lb Brussels sprouts
- 3 TBS balsamic vinegar
- 3 TBS olive oil

Sautee sprouts in olive oil on low heat until tender. Increase to high heat and add balsamic vinegar, stir for 30 seconds, turn off flame and season with salt to taste.

BAKED TILAPIA WITH LEMON AND FRESH HERBS

Servings: 4.

- 1 shallot, finely chopped
- 4 tilapia fillets
- 4 teaspoons olive oil
- sea salt
- 1 teaspoon finely chopped fresh thyme leaves
- ½ TBSP chopped parsley
- ½ TBSP fresh cilantro
- 1 teaspoon salt
- finely grated zest of 2 lemons

Mix herbs and seasonings with olive oil. Add Lemon zest and spread half of seasoning over fish. Place fish in broiler pan lined with parchment paper. Broil in pre-heated broiler for 3 minutes. Turn fish, applying remaining seasoning and broil for 3-5 minutes. Serve.

PORK TENDERLOIN

Servings: 6.

- 8 garlic cloves, coarsely chopped
- 1 tablespoon fresh oregano, finely chopped
- 1 tablespoon fresh thyme, finely chopped
- 1 tablespoon fresh rosemary, finely chopped
- 1 teaspoon salt
- 1/4 cup balsamic vinegar
- 1/2 cup olive oil
- 2 one pound pork tenderloins

Marinade pork for up to 24 hours in above ingredients.

Grill to perfection. Serve.

ROAST CHICKEN

Servings: 2-4.

- 1 whole chicken, 6 lbs.
- 1 lime, juiced
- 1/2 bunch cilantro
- 3 green onions, chopped
- 6 cloves garlic, peeled
- 1/4 cup olive oil
- 1 TBSP coconut oil
- salt

Chop and mix ingredients, rub chicken. Bake at 400 for 45 minutes.

GARLIC ROSEMARY SALMON

Servings: 2.

- 2 salmon fillets
- 5 cloves garlic, crushed
- olive oil - enough to coat the salmon
- dried rosemary to taste
- the juice from 1 lemon

Mix garlic with dill, olive oil, lemon and coat the salmon. Grill pan to perfection.

BEEF STEW

Servings: 4-6

- grass-fed beef brisket 3 Lbs.
- 10 garlic cloves, peeled
- salt to taste
- 1 bay leaf
- 1 ½ cups beef broth
- 8 cups of veggies leeks, carrots, celery, onions.

Cut slits into beef and add a peeled garlic clove in each. Sprinkle salt on beef. Chop up your veggies and add all ingredients to the slow cooker. Set on high for 4 hours or low for 8 hours.

CROCK POT CHICKEN

Servings : 6.

- 2.5 lbs boneless, skinless chicken thighs
- 3 parsnips
- 3 carrots
- 4 celery stalks
- 1 red onion
- 10-12 whole garlic cloves
- 1/4 cup coconut oil
- 1 cup chicken broth
- 1 TB fresh thyme
- 1 TB fresh sage
- Sea salt to taste

Add everything to your crock pot and let cook on high for 4 hours.

SAUTEED KALE

Servings: 4.

- 2 bunches of kale, leaves pulled off, discard stems
- 2 cloves garlic, finely chopped
- 1 TB olive oil

Sautee garlic in olive oil until golden brown, add in kale until tender.

GINGER SALMON AND BROCCOLI

Servings: 4.

- 1 head broccoli, cut into florets
- 2 TB coconut oil
- Sea salt
- 1 pound salmon
- squeeze of lemon
- ¼ bunch fresh cilantro
- 1 TBSP ginger, chopped
- 2 TBS coconut aminos

Cover salmon with coconut oil, cilantro, ginger, coconut aminos and a squeeze of lemon.

Grill pan to perfection and serve with steamed broccoli.

NORI CHIPS

Servings : 1.

- 3 Nori sheets
- olive oil
- sea salt

Preheat oven to 350. Cut Nori sheets into four and place on baking sheet. Brush or massage Nori with oil. Add sea salt and whatever spices you choose. Bake for 15 minutes. Let cool.

DESSERTS

Paleo Berry Ice Cream

Servings : 4.

1 pint of blueberries or your favorites

1/2 cup coconut milk

1 tsp vanilla extract

Blend everything in your food processor and place in freezer.

RASPBERRIES WITH BALSAMIC AND COCONUT MILK

Servings : 2.

- 40 Raspberries
- 2 TB balsamic vinegar
- coconut milk

Cover raspberries in a bowl with 2 TBS of balsamic and let sit for 15 minutes. Drizzle with coconut milk.

SNACKS

- Cucumber with sea salt
- Herbal tea
- Mixed fruit
- Coconut milk smoothie with plum, nectarine, peach, apple
- Nori Chips
- Kale Chips
- Coconut water kefir
- Coconut yogurt
- Avocado with sauerkraut
- Grated, Carrot, Daikon with Nori
- Bone Broth
- Veggie Broth

SUPER SONIC SALAD:

- 1 cup butter lettuce
- 1 cup spinach
- 1/2 cup dino kale (shredded)
- 1/4 cup parsley
- 1/8 cup fresh basil
- 1/8 cup carrots (diced or shredded)
- 1/8 cup celery (diced)

GINGER AVOCADO POWER DRESSING:

- 1/2 cup coconut or olive oil
- 1/3 cup raw apple cider vinegar
- 1/4 cup coconut aminos
- 1/2 cup water
- 2 tablespoon fresh ginger, grated
- 1 avocado

Blend and dress your salad!

BASIC BEEF BONE BROTH:

- 4 quarts water
- 2 lbs beef bones (or oxtail)
- 6 garlic cloves
- 3 ribs of celery
- 1 onion chopped
- 2 tablespoon apple cider vinegar
- 1 teaspoon sea salt

Place all ingredients in pot and bring the stock to a boil, then reduce the heat to low and allow the stock to cook from 8 hours. Allow the stock to cool then strain to discard bones etc. Store your stock in the fridge and use within a few days.

GINGER ROOT TEA:

- 4-6 cup filtered water
- 2 tab freshly grated ginger root
- 1 tablespoon fresh lemon juice

Bring ginger almost to boiling in the water. Turn off heat and let sit for 5-10 min. Add lemon juice and strain into a cup. You can reuse the ginger more than once by adding more water and heating.

Detox Support:Transitioning to The Autoimmune Paleo Plan

DETOX BATH RECIPE:

- 2 pounds of Epsom Salt plus
- 1 pound of baking soda
- 10 drops of lavender essential oil

DETOX BROTH:

- 3 quarts of water
- 1 large chopped onion
- 2 sliced carrots
- 1 cup of daikon
- 1 cup of turnips and rutabaga cut into large cubes
- 2 cups of chopped greens: kale, parsley, beet greens, collard greens, chard, dandelion, cilantro or other greens
- 2 celery stalks
- ½ cup of cabbage
- 4 ½ inch slices of ginger
- 2 cloves of whole garlic sea salt to taste

Add all the ingredients at once and place on low boil for 60 minutes. Cool and strain veggies out-discard them.

Makes approximately 8 cups. Store in fridge. Heat and drink 3-4 cups/day.

LIVER SUPPORT:

- olive oil & lemon juice (one tablespoon of each mixed with 4 oz. of water).

RAW APPLE CIDER VINEGAR:

1 tablespoon diluted with 1 tablespoon in water helps your stomach produce hydrochloric acid, and aid digestion of proteins.

EASY EXERCISE:

30 minute walk per day.

About the Author

Anne Angelone, Licensed Acupuncturist

Bachelor of Science, Cornell University Master of Science, American College of Traditional Chinese Medicine

Member of Primal Docs The Paleo Physician's Network

And Dr. Kharrazian's Thyroid Docs

✦ Background ✦

My own experience with Ankylosing Spondylitis (AS) led me to study the underlying mechanisms of disease expression. Since Ankylosing Spondylitis is correlated with the gene type called HLA B-27, I learned how to identify and remove specific triggers and then how to heal my leaky gut. I also learned how it's possible to turn off inflammatory gene expression with nutrition, supplements, Qi (oxygen), acupuncture, exercise, diet, and meditation. I'm grateful to be able to share what I have learned through experience and years of research, training and investigation.

My background in Functional Medicine has included advanced training with Dr. Datis Kharrazian in Functional Blood Chemistry Analysis, Mastering the Thyroid, Neurotransmitters and the Brain, Functional Endocrinology, Autoimmunity and Gluten Sensitivity

My hope is to share this information with those who would like to treat the underlying causes of "chronic symptoms" and experience greater health sooner than later

CONTINUING ALONG THE PATH OF HEALING:

Please help me spread the word about the simple yet profound equation for halting autoimmune reactions: remove triggers, resolve intestinal permeability and silence inflammatory gene expression. Please share this information with those who would like to treat the underlying causes of their "chronic symptoms".

If you would like to join an amazing group of people on the same healing path, head over to my website and check out the Autoimmune Paleo Challenge class page for more info and to participate in the next Autoimmune Paleo Challenge Tele-class.

For more info, please contact: www.anneangelone.com

AUTOIMMUNE PALEO RESOURCES:

- Sarah Ballantyne, Ph.D. aka: The Paleo Mom
- Autoimmune Paleo and You
- Autoimmune-Paleo
- Practical Paleo by Diane Sanfilippo And Balanced Bites
- Chris Kresser's: Personal Paleo Code
- The Paleo Parents Pinterest page
- Why Do I Still Have Thyroid Symptoms? When My Lab Tests Are Normal by Dr. Datis Kharrazian

The Paleo Approach: Reverse Autoimmune Disease and Heal Your Body by Sarah Ballantyne, PhD.

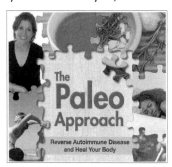

Made in the USA
San Bernardino, CA
22 October 2013